Zan Ferant
Nejc Kozar
Dusanka Micetic-Turk

Bone Mineral Density and Body Composition

AF153277

Zan Ferant
Nejc Kozar
Dusanka Micetic-Turk

Bone Mineral Density and Body Composition

Bone mineral density and body composition in children and adolescents with celiac disease and inflammatory bowel disease

LAP LAMBERT Academic Publishing

Impressum / Imprint

Bibliografische Information der Deutschen Nationalbibliothek: Die Deutsche Nationalbibliothek verzeichnet diese Publikation in der Deutschen Nationalbibliografie; detaillierte bibliografische Daten sind im Internet über http://dnb.d-nb.de abrufbar.

Alle in diesem Buch genannten Marken und Produktnamen unterliegen warenzeichen-, marken- oder patentrechtlichem Schutz bzw. sind Warenzeichen oder eingetragene Warenzeichen der jeweiligen Inhaber. Die Wiedergabe von Marken, Produktnamen, Gebrauchsnamen, Handelsnamen, Warenbezeichnungen u.s.w. in diesem Werk berechtigt auch ohne besondere Kennzeichnung nicht zu der Annahme, dass solche Namen im Sinne der Warenzeichen- und Markenschutzgesetzgebung als frei zu betrachten wären und daher von jedermann benutzt werden dürften.

Bibliographic information published by the Deutsche Nationalbibliothek: The Deutsche Nationalbibliothek lists this publication in the Deutsche Nationalbibliografie; detailed bibliographic data are available in the Internet at http://dnb.d-nb.de.

Any brand names and product names mentioned in this book are subject to trademark, brand or patent protection and are trademarks or registered trademarks of their respective holders. The use of brand names, product names, common names, trade names, product descriptions etc. even without a particular marking in this works is in no way to be construed to mean that such names may be regarded as unrestricted in respect of trademark and brand protection legislation and could thus be used by anyone.

Coverbild / Cover image: www.ingimage.com

Verlag / Publisher:
LAP LAMBERT Academic Publishing
ist ein Imprint der / is a trademark of
OmniScriptum GmbH & Co. KG
Heinrich-Böcking-Str. 6-8, 66121 Saarbrücken, Deutschland / Germany
Email: info@lap-publishing.com

Herstellung: siehe letzte Seite /
Printed at: see last page
ISBN: 978-3-659-58499-2

TABLE OF CONTENTS

1 INTRODUCTION 3

1.1 CELIAC DISEASE 3

1.2 INFLAMMATORY BOWEL DISEASE (IBD) 6

1.2.1 Ulcerative colitis (UC) 7

1.2.2 Crohn's disease 8

1.3 CELIAC DISEASE, INFLAMMATORY BOWEL DISEASE AND BONE MINERAL DENSITY 10

1.3.1 RANK-RANKL-OPG pathway 11

1.3.2 Vitamin D 12

2 AIMS AND HYPOTHESES 14

3 PATIENTS AND METHODS 15

3.1 PATIENTS 15

3.2 METHODS 16

3.2.1 Dual-energy X-ray absorptiometry (DXA) 16

3.2.2 Bone age 16

3.2.3 Vitamin D 17

3.2.4 Serological markers 17

3.2.5 Bioimpedance analysis (BIA) 18

3.2.6 Statistical methods 18

4 RESULTS 19

5 DISCUSSION 30

5.1 BONE MINERAL DENSITY AND BONE AGE 30

5.2 VITAMIN D 32

5.3 BODY COMPOSITION 34

5.4 SEROLOGIC MARKERS 35

6 CONCLUSION 38

7 REFERENCES 39

8 ACKNOWLEDGEMENTS 52

TABLE OF FIGURES AND TABLES

Figure 1: RANK-RANKL-OPG pathway 12

Figure 2: Multifactoral cause of lowered BMD 13

Table 1: Patients by sex and age in different groups 19

Table 2: BMD and bone age in different groups... 19

Figure 3: Lumbar spine BMD in different groups. 20

Figure 4: Left hip BMD in different groups.. 21

Figure 5: Mean serum vitamin D in different groups. 22

Figure 6: Percentage of body fat (BF %) in different groups (divided by sex). 23

Figure 7: LBM in different groups (divided by sex)... 24

Figure 8: BMD in t-TG negative and positive CD patients. 26

Figure 9: BMD in EMA negative and positive CD patients. 27

Figure 10: Lumbar spine BMD in serologically negative CD patients....................... 28

Figure 11: Left hip BMD in serologically negative CD patients................................. 29

1 INTRODUCTION

Studies have shown increased incidence of lowered bone mineral density (BMD) in children and adolescents with celiac disease (CD) or inflammatory bowel disease (IBD). However, exact pathogenetic mechanisms are not entirely known (1-11). Changes in BMD are reversible; they improve with treatment, i. e. gluten-free diet (GFD) in patients with CD and specific treatment in patients with IBD (2-5,8). The aim of our research was to explore the prevalence of lowered BMD in children and adolescents with CD and IBD in NE Slovenia. In addition, we expanded our research by determining patients' bone age and vitamin D values. We also investigated possible effect of patients' body composition (measured with bioelectrical impedance analysis - BIA) on BMD. We determined the usefulness of BIA, which represents a handy and patient-friendly method. To further explore BMD in CD patients, we measured their CD serologic markers (endomysial antibodies - EMA and antibodies against tissue ransglutaminase - t-TG) in attempt to quantify strictness of their GFD.

1.1 CELIAC DISEASE

CD is an immune-mediated systemic disorder elicited by gluten and related prolamines in genetically susceptible individuals and characterised by the presence of a variable combination of gluten-dependent clinical manifestations, CD-specific antibodies, HLA-DQ2 or HLA-DQ8 haplotypes, and enteropathy (12).

Prevalence of CD in European and US pediatric population is approaching 1% (13,14). Even though European and US data are comparable, latest studies show increase of prevalence of CD in European countries (15,16). In other countries CD is not diagnosed as well as it is in Europe or US, but prevalence of CD is thought to be comparable. Exception is Subsaharan Africa, where it has been reported, that the prevalence of CD can also reach up to 5% (17).

The presence of gluten in small intestines is essential for causing epithelial damage in genetically susceptible individuals. Peptides like gliadin, are penetrating between epithelium, where they are deaminated with the help of tissue transglutaminase (t-TG). Deamination enables binding to HLA-DQ2 and DQ8 receptors on T lymphocytes, which activate cytotoxic T cells in that way stimulating epithelium injury and formation of antibodies typical for CD (18).

Complex link between genetic and environmental factors is typical of the disease, which manifests itself as enteropathy with malabsorption of nutrients and vitamins (19,20). It has been demonstrated that some gliadin peptides resistant to complete proteolytic digestion may directly affect intestinal cell structure and functions by modulating gene expression and oxidative stress (21).

Clinical features of CD are very diverse. We can still observe classic clinical feature of small hypothonic uninterested child with enlarged abdomen and steatorrhea. However, nowadays most patients manifest with mild symptoms or they are diagnosed as a result of screening (22). Children present with mostly gastrointestinal and malnutritional symtoms. In addition, skin, liver, central nervous system, lung and other organs can represent primary affected organ (23). Children can also manifest with extraintestinal symptoms or symptoms which are linked to malabsorption. These include stunted growth, anemia and lowered BMD (24).

Reduced BMD is frequently found in individuals with celiac CD, who are not consuming a GFD, possibly due to calcium and vitamin D malabsorption, release of pro-inflammatory cytokines, and misbalanced bone remodeling (25).

The prevalence of CD among first-degree relatives is much higher than the prevalence of the disease in the general population. Most of these patients have an atypical presentation of the disease and would be therefore overlooked without an active search (26). CD is strongly associated with HLA-DQ2 and/or HLA-DQ8, as both genotypes predispose for the disease development (27,28). For that reason, serological testing is recommended for all first-degree relatives of CD patients. In addition, they should undergo HLA typing to detect those whose HLA phenotype is consistent with CD. This approach can also help in excluding individuals who do not need further diagnostic procedures (26). Currently, serological screening tests are primarily utilized to identify those individuals in need of a diagnostic endoscopic biopsy, although there is a possibility to diagnose the disease solely based on serology according to latest guidelines of European Society for Paediatric Gastroenterology, Hepatology and Nutrition (ESPGHAN) (12). Ultrasonography may also provide valuable information on small-bowel wall structure and can help in decision making on the necessity of small bowel biopsy. However, there is a much stronger correlation between serological markers and CD then between ultrasonography and CD (29,30). The determination of serum levels of t-TG antibodies is the first choice in screening for celiac disease (12).

Enteroscopy examination for CD should be reserved for patients with positive serology and negative histopathology at initial esophagogastroduodenoscopy, and in the search for complications during a follow-up. Enteroscopy cannot be recommended at the initial work-up of CD patients (31).

Tissue transglutaminase is a crucial factor in CD because it promotes the gluten-specific T-cell response and is also the target of the autoimmune response. Tissue transglutaminase induces changes in gluten, which in turn, causes the generation of a series of gluten peptides that bind to HLA-DQ2 or DQ8 molecules with high affinity. The resulting HLA-DQ2 HLA-DQ8-gluten peptide interaction triggers the proinflammatory T cell response. Tissue transglutaminase is also involved in other non-T-cell-mediated biological activities of gliadin peptides (32). In addition, the anti-endomisial antibodies (EMA) are frequently used in the diagnosis of CD, and positive EMA is a very strong predictor of a disease (33,34). Once the diagnosis has been established, serological testing is being routinely used in the monitoring of the response to a GFD (12,35,36). There is evidence that decreased concentrations of antibodies are significantly associated with the degree of compliance with the GFD. Among others, t-TG has the best and most consistent performances. The serial measurement of antibody levels seems to be more reliable in monitoring compliance than the positive/negative expression of results (37,38). Periodical serological and

5

clinical follow-ups are a viable and efficient strategy to promote adherence to gluten-free diet (39,40). Measuring EMA and t-TG is recommended every 12 months (41).

The only efficient treatment of CD at the moment consists of a strict, lifelong GFD, which promotes an improvement of the disease activity which yields to the recovery of bone mineralization in children (25,42). Studies confirmed the significance of compliance with GFD in children with CD until the end of bone mineralization even in asymptomatic patients (4,5,43). It is virtually impossible to sustain GFD without any gluten, because food is often contaminated with gluten. Additionally, the presence of wheat in production facilities could contaminate cereals and other otherwise gluten-free foodstuffs (51). That is why foodstuffs in GFD are those which are tolerated by most CD patients. With increased sensitivity of methods for determining traces of gluten in foodstuffs the allowed threshold of gluten changes. Codex Alimentarius from 2008 dictates the threshold is at 20 mg gluten/kg foodstuff. In this order, patients on strict GFD ingest less than 10mg of gluten daily (45). Strict GFD improves bone mineralization, while raising of BMD can be observed as quick as the first year after implementing GFD (3,46).

1.2 INFLAMMATORY BOWEL DISEASE (IBD)

IBD is a group of diseases with unknown etiology. They are chronic, usually lifelong diseases with acute relapses and remissions. IBD is characterized by severe inflammation of the small bowel and/or colon leading to recurrent diarrhea and persistent abdominal pain. Crohn's disease and ulcerative colitis (UC) are two main clinicopathological subtypes of IBD. Patients who cannot be classified as neither of those two subtypes are diagnosed as indeterminate colitis (47).

Incidence of UC and Crohn's disease in Slovenia is 5/100,000 and 3,6/100,000, respectively (47). IBD is distributed bimodally with early onset between ages of 10 and 20 and second peak between age 50 and 80. 25% of patients are diagnosed before the age of 20. Disease can present itself in as early as one year olds and in the last

6

decade we can observe increased incidence in pediatric population (mostly due to Crohn's disease) (48).

Pathogenesis of IBD consists of genetic and environmental factors. Environmental factors are important in IBD pathogenesis and could explain discordance in twins and within the same race in different geographic regions. However, exact factors remain unknown. Individuals who immigrate to more developed countries are exposed to higher risk for IBD. The most important factor in IBD pathogenesis is supposed to be immunoregulation of intestinal mucosa. Genetic vulnerability leads to disrupted identification and presentation of intestinal antigens to effector cells. Mechanism that controls and limits this inflammation does not work correctly in IBD and allows for pathologic inflammation. Whether the inflammation is abnormal response to usual intestinal antigens or normal response to unknown microbe remains to be confirmed (48,49).

1.2.1 Ulcerative colitis (UC)

UC is chronic inflammatory disease involving the colon, and is an important cause of chronic gastrointestinal disease in children and adolescents. Disease usually begins in the rectum and extends proximally for a variable distance. Blood in the stool and diarrhea are the typical presentation of UC. Symptoms such as tenesmus, urgency, cramping abdominal pain (especially with bowel movements), and nocturnal bowel movements are common (47,48).

It is generally believed that the risk of colon cancer begins to increase after 8 – 10 years of disease and may then increase by 0.5 – 1 % per year. Because colon cancer is usually preceded by changes of mucosal dysplasia, it is recommended that patients who have had UC for more than 10 years be screened with colonoscopy and biopsy every 1 – 2 years (48).

The diagnosis of UC must be confirmed by endoscopic and histologic examination of the colon. Classically, the disease starts in the rectum with a gross appearance characterized by erythema, edema, loss of vascular pattern, granularity, and friability. Inflammation is limited to mucosa and sometimes to submucosa. There may be a "cutoff" demarcating the margin between inflammation and normal colon, or the entire colon may be involved (48).

Treatment of UC is aimed at controlling symptoms and reducing the risk of recurrence. 20 – 30 % of individuals with UC have spontaneous improvement in symptoms. Oral sulfasalazine is usually effective in the treatment of mild colitis. Children with moderate to severe pancolitis or colitis should be treated with corticosteroids, most commonly, prednisone. Prolonged use of daily steroids beyond this period is to be avoided because of the many side effects, including growth retardation, adrenal suppression, cataracts, osteopenia among others. Budenoside, a newer corticosteroid, has limited systemic effects. Many children with disease requiring frequent corticosteroid therapy are started on immunosuppressive therapy such as azathioprine and/or 6-mercaptopurine. Cyclosporine is useful in children with acute steroid refractory UC. Infliximab, a chimeric monoclonal antibody to tumor necrosis factor–α (TNF- α), has been used in some cases of fulminant UC. Colectomy is performed for intractable disease, complications of therapy, and fulminant disease that is unresponsive to medical management (47,48).

1.2.2 Crohn's disease

Crohn's disease, an idiopathic, chronic inflammatory disorder of the bowel, involves any region of the alimentary tract from the mouth to the anus. The inflammatory process tends to be eccentric and segmental, often with skip areas (normal regions of bowel between inflamed areas). Although inflammation in UC is limited to the mucosa (except in toxic megacolon), gastrointestinal involvement in Crohn's disease is transmural (48).

Patients with small bowel disease are more likely to have an obstructive pattern (most commonly with right lower quadrant pain), while those with colonic disease are more likely to have symptoms resulting from inflammation (diarrhea, bleeding, cramping). Fever, malaise, and easy fatiguability are common. Growth failure with delayed bone maturation and delayed sexual development may precede other symptoms by 1 or 2 years and is at least twice as likely to occur with Crohn's disease as with UC. Extraintestinal manifestations occur more commonly with Crohn's disease than with UC; those that are especially associated with Crohn's disease include oral aphthous ulcers, peripheral arthritis, erythema nodosum, digital clubbing, episcleritis, renal stones (uric acid, oxalate), and gallstones. In contrast to UC, perianal disease is common (tags, fistula, abscess) (48).

The small and large bowel should be examined in the child with suspected Crohn's disease. Linear ulcers may give a cobblestone appearance to the mucosal surface. Diseased regions tend to be eccentric while normal regions may be found between diseased segments (skip areas) (48).

The medical treatment for a child with Crohn's disease should be individualized based on the degree and site of intestinal involvement, extraintestinal manifestation and nutritional status (50). Inflammation responds to corticosteroids better than to aminosalicylates. However, growth is impaired with either active disease or daily corticosteroid therapy. Nutritional deficiencies due to suboptimal caloric intakes, malabsorption, or increased losses are common in children with Crohn's disease. Therefore, enteral nutrition with semielemental or elemental formulae are used to optimize calories intake. The use of sulfasaliazine and mesalamine, antibiotics such as metronidazole and ciprofloxacil and immunosuppressive therapy as 6-mercaptopurine and azathioprine, methotrexate and cyclosporine and tacrolimus are the drugs that are used for in the treatment of children and adolescents with different stages of the disease. Infliximab, a chimeric monoclonal antibody to TNF-α, has been approved for the initial treatment and subsequent maintenance therapy of adults with Crohn disease. It is commonly used in children, and noncontrolled published series suggest marked symptom improvement in 50 − 70% of patients. Surgical therapy should be reserved for specific indications; recurrence rate after bowel resection is high (more than 50 % by fifth year) (49,51).

Psychosocial issues for the child with Crohn's disease include a sense of being different, concerns about body image, difficulty in not participating fully in age-appropriate activities, and family conflict brought on by the added stress of this disease. Patients who are socially "connected" fare better. Ongoing education about the disease is an important aspect of management because children generally fare better if they understand and anticipate problems (49,52).

Crohn's disease is a chronic disorder that is associated with high morbidity but low mortality (49). Weight loss and growth failure can usually be improved with treatment and attention to nutritional needs. Osteopenia is particularly common in those with chronic poor nutrition and frequent exposure to high doses of corticosteroids. The region of bowel involved may increase with time, although rapid progression typically occurs early and is subsequently slow. The risk of colon cancer in individuals with long-standing Crohn's colitis approaches that associated with UC and screening colonoscopy is indicated after 10 years of colonic disease. Despite these complications, most children with Crohn's disease lead active, full lives with only intermittent flare-up in symptoms (48).

1.3 CELIAC DISEASE, INFLAMMATORY BOWEL DISEASE AND BONE MINERAL DENSITY

Chronic inflammatory gastrointestinal diseases like CD and IBD are known to cause alterations in bone metabolism (1-11). Without therapy and strict GFD, CD is associated with malabsorption of calcium and vitamin D, which reduces serum calcium and stimulates the release of parathormone, thereby exacerbating bone reabsorption from the mobilization of bone calcium (53-56). This progressively leads to a decrease in BMD that, in turn, can lead to osteopenia or even osteoporosis with possible devastating complications in later life (57-60). Over 75 % of untreated patients with CD have low BMD (61). However, a GFD improves bone mineralization, already within the first year of treatment (3-5).

Children with IBD gain bone mass, but the rate of bone mineral accrual is slower than in their healthy peers, at least during the first 2 years after the diagnosis (56). It is reasonable to hypothesize that decreases in the rate of bone accrual may lead to suboptimal peak bone mass which is known to be reached in the third decade of life (62-64). Catch-up growth may not occur in children with IBD, and inadequate linear growth may stunt the normal acquisition of bone minerals (56). For that reason, these young adults could be in a disadvantageous position regarding their bone health in later life, possibly resulting in symptomatic osteoporosis (62,64). There are several possible mechanisms of IBD-related reduction of BMD, including malabsorption and malnutrition, prolonged corticosteroid therapy, restriction diets that are low in vitamin D and calcium, and also immobilization (8,65). In recent years, the role of inflammation is becoming more and more important in the pathogenesis of reduced BMD (8,61,66,67).

1.3.1 RANK-RANKL-OPG pathway

A new TNF family pathway involved in bone metabolism, known as the RANK-RANKL-OPG pathway, has been described (68). RANKL (receptor-activator of NFκB ligand) is expressed on the surface of osteoblasts, synovial stromal cells and activated T cells. RANKL binds to either osteoclast precursors expressing the RANKL receptor (receptor-activator of NFκB – RANK) or a soluble decoy receptor osteoprotegerin (OPG), which is produced by osteoblasts. If RANKL and RANK interact, osteoclasts differentiate and mature, resulting in increased bone loss. OPG blocks this interaction, thereby inhibiting osteoclast production. Compounds such as parathyroid hormone (PTH), $1\alpha,25$-(OH)2D3 (calcitriol – active form of vitamin D), prostaglandin E2 and dexamethasone stimulate RANKL expression and inhibit OPG production, thereby causing increased osteoclastogenesis, whereas 17β-estradiol increases OPG and decreases RANKL, reducing osteoclastogenesis (66,68) (Figure

11

1). The small bowel of patients with CD contains a marked increase in intraepithelial and lamina propria lymphocytes, potentially releasing cytokines that alter the balance of the RANK-RANKL paradigm toward osteoclastogenesis (69,70). Recent clinical studies in patients with IBD have revealed that serum OPG levels may be elevated and that inflamed intestinal tissue secretes increased amounts of OPG. It is suspected that OPG levels are elevated as a counterregulatory response to low BMD, as serum OPG levels in IBD have been found to be inversely associated with BMD (71).

Figure 1: RANK-RANKL-OPG pathway

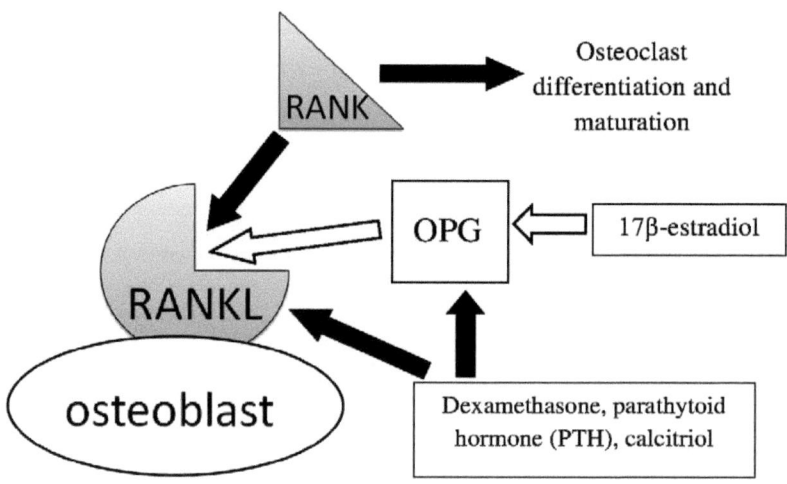

Figure 1 shows binding of either RANK or OPG on ligand RANKL. Black arrows represent factors that increase osteoclastogenesis and thus bone loss while white arrows represent factors which reduce osteoclastogenesis.

1.3.2 Vitamin D

Patients with CD and IBD are at higher risk for vitamin D deficiency. Decreased exposure to sunlight, decreased dietary intake, malabsorption and gastrointestinal loss may all well contribute to lowered serum levels of vitamin (62,72-75). The loss of albumin as the binding protein for vitamin D is well documented in patients with IBD, and may also be a risk factor that contributes to the pathology of disease (76).

To avoid complications in the future, like impaired growth, suboptimal peak bone mass or risk of fractures, it is important to diagnose and treat complications of chronic inflammatory gastrointestinal diseases.

Figure 2: Multifactoral cause of lowered BMD

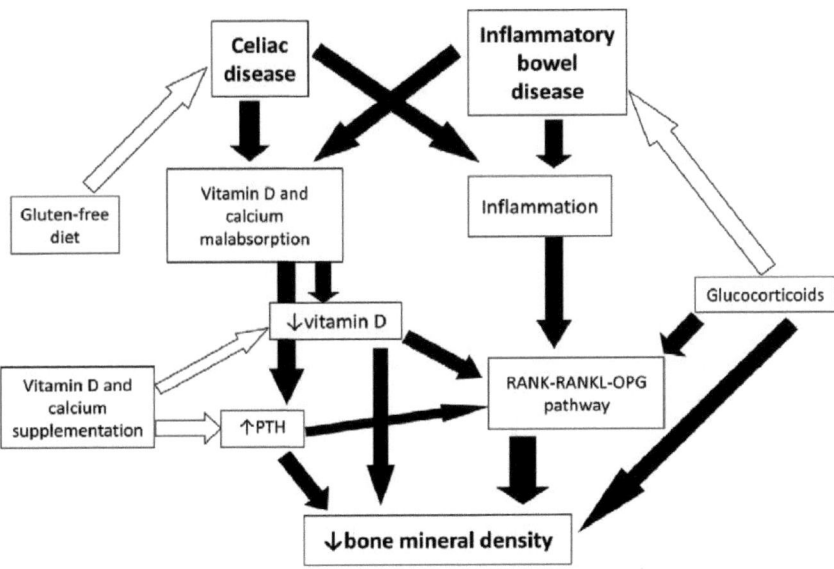

Figure shows intricate mechanism of lowered BMD in CD and IBD. White arrows represent factors that improve disease and help maintain normal BMD, while black arrows represent factors that lower BMD.

2 AIMS AND HYPOTHESES

The aim of this study was to asses BMD in pediatric patients with CD, IBD and healthy control group, to determine levels of vitamin D in these groups and to asses the value of BIA as a diagnostic tool in diagnosing lowered BMD.

Our goal was to verify next hypotheses:

1. BMD in patients with CD and IBD is significantly lower than BMD in healthy controls.
2. Values of vitamin D in patients with CD and IBD are significantly lower than vitamin D values in healthy controls.
3. BIA results correlate with BMD; therefore BIA is a useful method in diagnosing lowered BMD.

Additionally, we assesed the following parameters:

4. Compliance with strict GFD in our group of CD patients (measured with serologic markers EMA and t-TG).
5. Correlation of serologic markers (EMA and t-TG) values with BMD.
6. Bone age in different groups.

3 PATIENTS AND METHODS

3.1 PATIENTS

In this prospective case controlled study, which was conducted between March 2011 and April 2012, a total of 113 children aged between 10 and 18 years were selected and followed-up. They were divided into three different groups: children with CD (n = 41; 18 boys, 23 girls), children with IBD (n = 35; 19 boys, 16 girls) and a healthy control group (n = 37; 19 boys, 18 girls). All patients with CD were previously diagnosed according to the diagnostic criteria of the European Society for Paediatric Gastroenterology, Hepatology and Nutrition (ESPGHAN), which includes histological demonstration of villous atrophy in duodenal mucosa and positive serological markers (12). Even though all of the CD patients declared to be on a strict GFD during the period of at least 6 months before the study. IBD patients were receiving appropriate treatment and were all in stable remission for at least 6 months prior to the study. IBD patients were also given calcium and vitamin D supplements and were advised to take them regularly. They did not receive any corticosteroid treatment during the period of the study. After initial diagnosis was established and written consent obtained from parents or children if they were old enough, children and adolescents were included in the study. None of our patients had any bone or joint pain or any history of lowered BMD.

The control group consisted of healthy children and adolescents who showed no symptoms of CD or IBD and who came to the Pediatric Clinic for their check-ups following their hospitalization due to a particular health condition such as pneumonia, urinary tract infection, otitis media, diarrhoea, etc. Nine subjects from control group were voluntarily recruited from the general population and the rest of the subjects in control group had no previous or present suspicion of a chronic gastrointestinal disorder. During their visit, parent(s) and child/adolescent received information regarding the study. After obtaining their written consent, participants

15

were included in the study and all necessary measurements were taken by trained medical personnel.

Patients with CD and IBD were invited to participate during their regular follow-up visits. Two participants with CD, however, did not reach inclusion criteria and were consequently excluded form the study. The reasons for exclusion were hypertension (1 adolescent) and chronic kidney disease (1 adolescent). In addition, 7 patients with CD, 3 with IBD and 8 subjects from control group agreed to participate but after clinical and laboratory work-up they did not complete the appointed DXA measurement. All participants included in the study were Caucasians residing in North-Eastern Slovenia. The study was approved by the Slovene National Medical Ethics Committee.

3.2 METHODS

3.2.1 Dual-energy X-ray absorptiometry (DXA)

BMD was measured at lumbar spine (L1-L4) and left hip in 97 patients using dual-energy X-ray absorptiometry (Hologic Explorer QDR). The device and the system were calibrated daily. BMD was expressed as Z-score, which is the number of standard deviations above or below the mean for the patient's age, sex and ethnicity and is determined from local reference data; not to be confused with T-score, which is standard deviation unit used in relation to the young healthy population and it is used in expressing DXA results in adults (46).

3.2.2 Bone age

Bone or skeletal age was determined in all participants in order to assess their chronological bone development. X-ray imaging and interpretation were conducted on left hand and wrist at the Department of Radiology at University Medical Centre Maribor using standard radiological doctrine. Bone age was then compared to chronological age of the patient and result was expressed as the difference between the two, where positive difference indicated that bone age precedes chronological age of patient.

3.2.3 Vitamin D

Vitamin D measurements were conducted at the Department of laboratory diagnostics, University Medical Centre Maribor, Slovenia. Serum vitamin D levels were determined in all the patients and healthy controls with standard methods (Cobas, Roche). Normal range of serum vitamin D is between 47.7 and 144 nmol/L (19.1 – 57.6 ng/ml).

3.2.4 Serological markers

Antibodies against tissue transglutaminase were measured by Department of laboratory diagnostics at University Medical Centre Maribor using standardized methods (Luminex, AtheNA Multi-Lyte® Celiac Plus Assay, The Zeus Scientific). Cut-off values were 100 U/ml, where higher values were considered positive. According to manufacturer, the sensitivity and specifity of IgA antibodies against t-TG were 93.1 % and 77.3 %, respectively (77). This method was used at our University Medical Centre until 2012 when it was replaced by Eu-tTg IgA (Eurospital). Sensitivity of the test is 99.2 % and specificity 98.7 %. Reference limits issued by manufacturer of test are ‹ 9.0 U/ml for negative, borderline between 9.0 U/ml and 16.0 U/ml and positive 16.0 U/ml.

IgA antiendomysial antibodies were also determined at the Department of laboratory diagnostics at University Medical Centre Maribor using standardized flourescent method (Antiendomysium 96, Eurospital). Results were interpreted as positive or negative by medical personnel. As stated in studies by manufacturer, sensitivity of IgA antibodies against antiendomysium was 98 % and specificity was 99 % (78).

3.2.5 Bioimpedance analysis (BIA)

BIA is a fast, non-invasive and painless method. It (QuadScan 4000, Bodystat Ltd., Douglas, Isle of Man) was used in our study to determine percentage of body fat (BF %) and lean body mass (LBM, measured in kg). Measurements were conducted at Gastroenterology Unit, Department of Paediatrics at University Medical Centre in Maribor. All our subjets were fasting and were appropriately hidrated. Children's and adolescents' anthropometric measurements – body height (cm), waist circumference (cm) and body weight (kg) – were collected by medical personnel using standardized procedures. Measurements were conducted with our subjects lying in supine position on a flat, nonconductive bed. Bodystat QuadScan 4000 has four electrodes. Two electrodes were placed on the right wrist with one just proximal to the third metacarpophalangeal joint (positive) and one on the wrist next to the ulnar head (negative). The other two electrodes were placed on the right ankle with one just proximal to the third metatarsophalangeal joint (positive) and one between the medial and lateral malleoli (negative). Multifrequency (5, 50, 100, and 200 kHz) currents were introduced from the positive leads and traveled throughout the body to the negative leads. BF % was calculated by using the manufacturer's software.

3.2.6 Statistical methods

SPSS v. 16.0.1 statistical package for Windows was used to perform statistical analysis. Graphs were plotted to illustrate the relation between means of certain results. ANOVA test was used to determine statistical significance.

18

4 RESULTS

Table 1: Patients by sex and age in different groups

	CD		IBD		Control group		Total
Sex	Male	Female	Male	Female	Male	Female	113
Gender (%)	18 (44 %)	23 (56 %)	19 (54 %)	16 (46 %)	19 (51 %)	18 (49 %)	100 %
Mean age (years)	14.7	13.6	15.7	15.4	13.5	13.9	14.5

113 children aged between 10 and 18 years were divided into three different groups: children with CD (n = 41), children with IBD (n = 35) and healthy group (n = 37).

Table 2: BMD and bone age in different groups

Diagnosis	Lumbar spine BMD [Z score]	Left hip BMD [Z score]	Bone age [difference in yrs]
CD	- 0.2	- 0.4	0.2
IBD	- 0.4	- 0.6	0.1
Control group	- 0.3	- 0.8	0.2
P value	0.450	0.215	0.820

Bone age is expressed as difference in years between bone and chronological age. Positive values indicate that bone age precedes chronological age.

When comparing the mean lumbar spine BMD Z scores for two test groups we found that the CD patients had mean Z values of BMD of – 0.2, which is similar to the control group (- 0.3) (Table 1). Patients with IBD had mean lumbar spine BMD Z score was - 0.4 (Figure 3). BMD Z scores measured at lumbar spine in patients with CD, patients with IBD and control group did not differ significantly (p = 0.450).

Figure 3: Lumbar spine BMD in different groups.

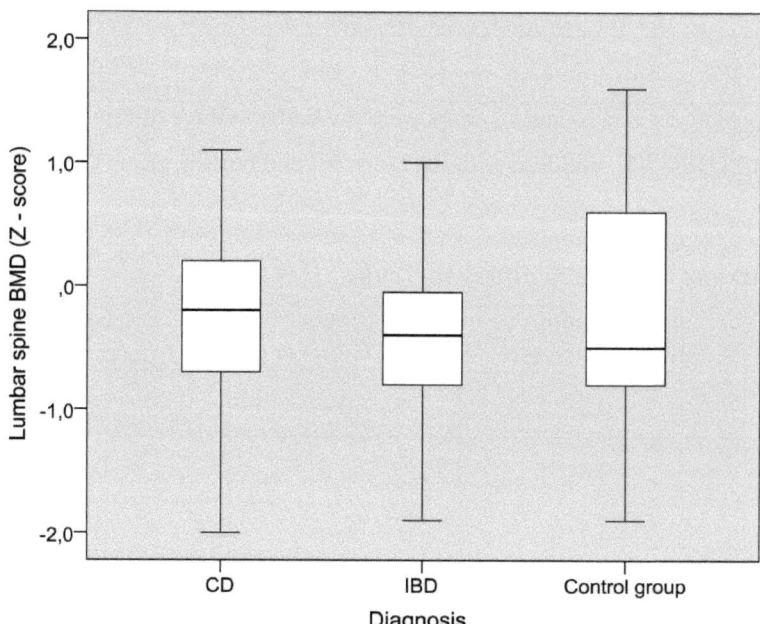

Figure shows comparison of lumbar spine BMD Z scores between different groups. BMD Z scores measured at lumbar spine in patients with CD, patients with IBD and control group do not differ significantly (p = 0.450).

After analyzing the mean left hip BMD Z scores for two test groups we observed a similar distribution of measured data. Mean left hip BMD Z score of CD patients was - 0.4, compared to - 0.8 in control group (- 0.8). IBD patients had mean Z scores of - 0.6 (Figure 4). The mean BMD Z scores were calculated in all patients in CD group, regardless of the strictness of their GFD. However, differences in left hip BMD Z scores between groups did not show statistical significance (p = 0.215).

Figure 4: Left hip BMD in different groups.

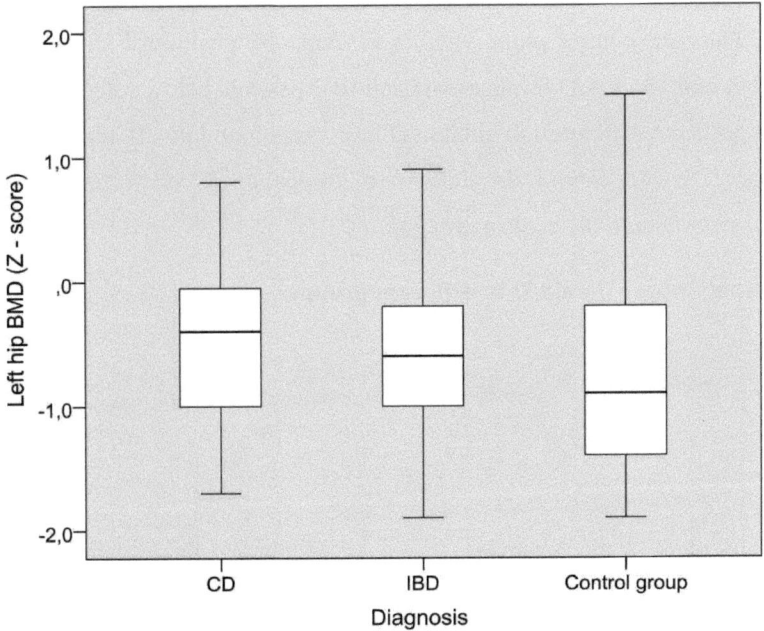

Figure shows comparison of left hip BMD Z scores between different groups. BMD Z scores measured at left hip in patients with CD, patients with IBD and control group do not differ significantly (p = 0.215).

Bone age or bone development was assessed by comparing the difference in bone and chronological age in different groups of patients. Mean bone and chronological age difference was 0.2 years for patients with CD, 0.1 years for IBD patients and 0.2 years for subjects in control group. Positive values of the difference between bone and chronological age represent that bone age precedes chronological age. There was no statistically significant difference between the groups (p = 0.820).

When measuring serum vitamin D levels, the mean vitamin D levels of 32.5 nmol/L in CD patients was observed. Mean vitamin D levels of IBD patients was similar with 32.6 nmol/L. Control group had the highest measured levels of vitamin D (49.9 nmol/L). Reference values used at our University Medical Centre range from 47.7 to 144 nmol/L. Thus our control group vitamin D levels are positioned slightly above the lower limit, and vitamin D levels of CD and IBD patients below reference values (Figure 5). Significant difference in vitamin D levels was found in CD and IBD group when compared to the control. In those two groups levels of vitamin D were significantly lower than in the control group ($p < 0.01$).

Figure 5: Mean serum vitamin D in different groups.

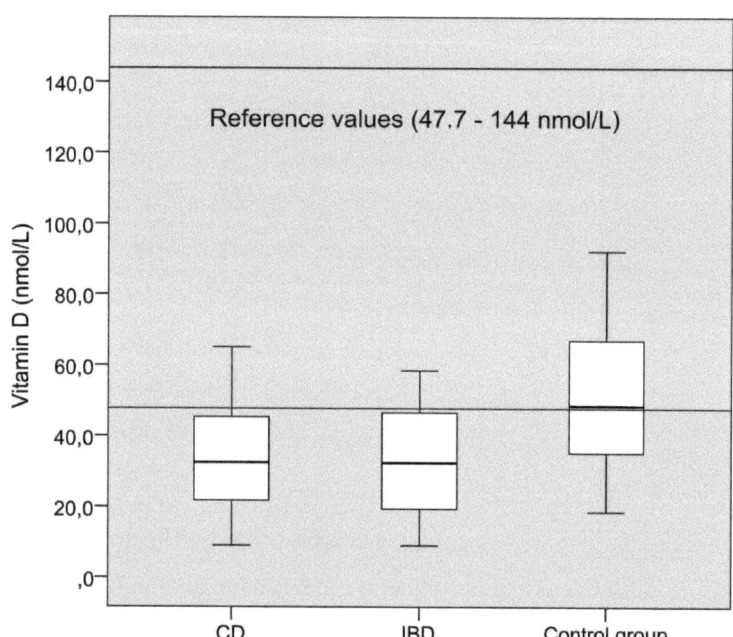

Significant difference ($p < 0.01$) in mean vitamin D levels was found in patients with CD and IBD when compared to the control group. Mean vitamin D level in control group was within the reference values with 49.9 nmol/L. The serum vitamin D levels were decreased with mean value of 32.5 nmol/L for CD patients and 32.6 nmol/L for IBD patients.

Within groups children were divided by sex, because percentage of their body fat (BF %) differed anthropometrically. Boys with CD had mean BF % of 13.8 (n = 12), boys with IBD had mean BF % of 20.7 (n = 14) and boys in control group had mean BF % of 18.0 (n = 18) (Figure 6). Girls had mean BF % values higher than boys. Mean BF % of CD girls was 22.1 (n = 17), mean BF % of IBD girls was 26.9 (n = 12), and mean BF % of girls in control group was 26.5 (n = 19). BF % did not differ significantly between the groups (p = 0.201 and p = 0.134 for boys and girls, respectively).

Figure 6: Percentage of body fat (BF %) in different groups (divided by sex).

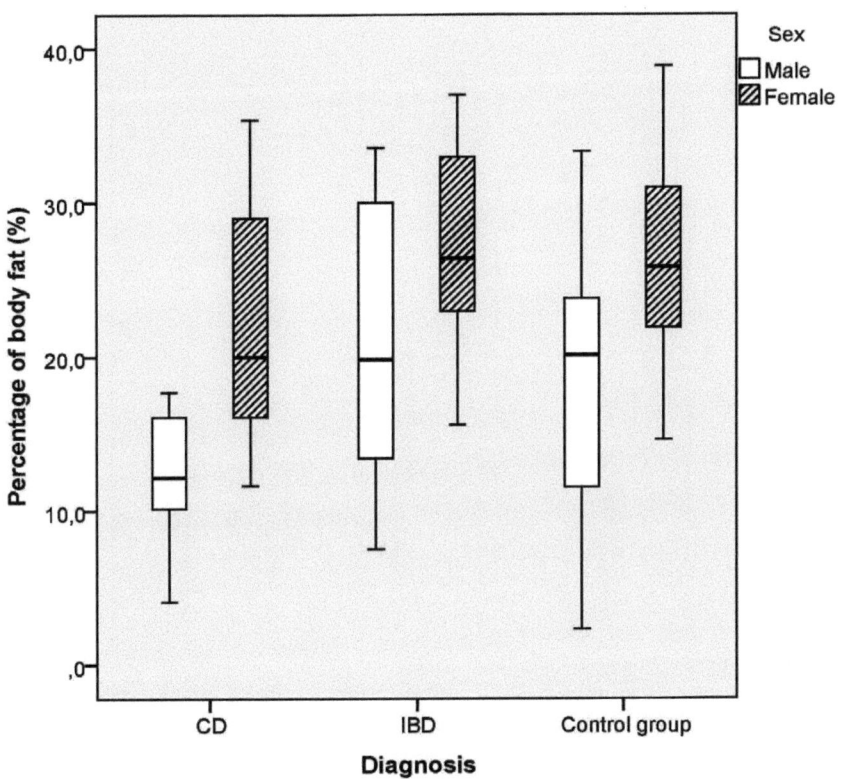

Figure shows comparison in BF % in CD patients, IBD patients and control group. Patients were divided by sex. Empty bars represent boys and bars with slanted black lines represent girls. BF % did not differ significantly (p = 0.201 in boys and p = 0.134 in girls).

The mean lean body mass (LBM) in boys with CD was 51.4 (n = 12), boys with IBD 49.6 (n = 14), boys in control group had mean LBM of 44.5 (n = 18) (Figure 7). Girls with CD had mean LBM of 34.2 (n = 15), girls with IBD 47.1 (n = 12) and girls in control group had mean LBM of 38.3 (n = 19). All measurements are expressed in kilograms. LBM did not differ significantly between the groups of boys (p = 0.262) but we found statistical significant difference between groups of girls (p = 0.007).

Figure 7: LBM in different groups (divided by sex).

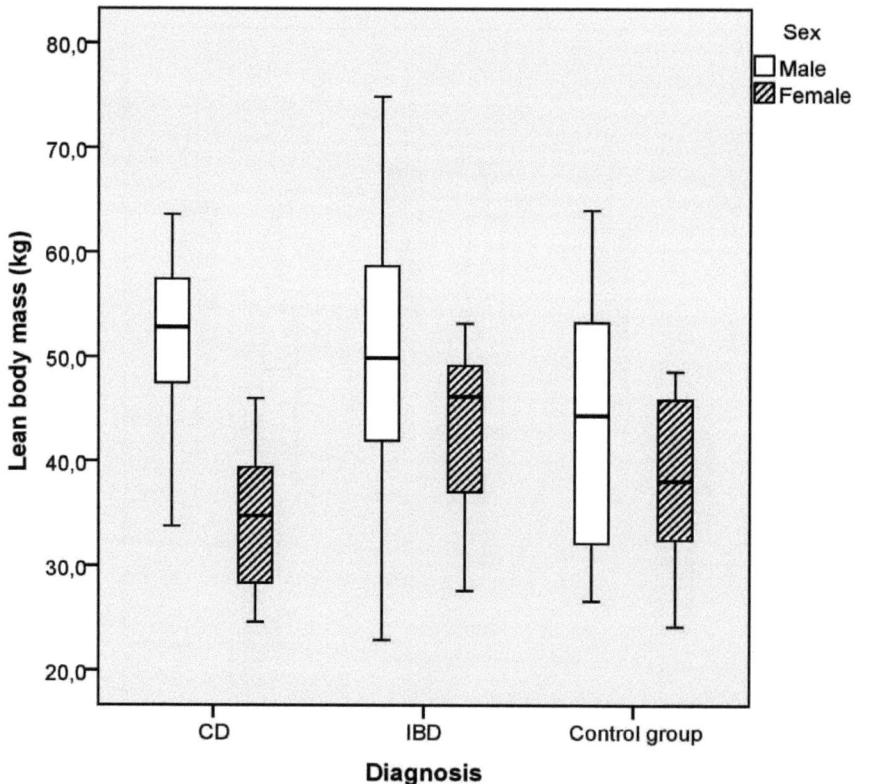

Figure shows comparison in LBM in CD patients, IBD patients and control group. Patients were divided by sex. Empty bars represent boys and bars with slanted black lines represent girls. LBM did not differ significantly in boys (p = 0.262) but it did in girls (p = 0.007).

Furthermore, our results showed no correlation between BF % and BMD Z scores. We compared all of our patient groups, divided by sex, but also all together. None of our comparisons with lumbar spine or left hip BMD Z scores were statistically significant. That was also the case when comparing LBM with BMD Z scores in all groups of patients.

Even though all patients included in the present study declared to be on a GFD for the period of at least six months prior to the study; 44 % of children and adolescents from the study were serologically positive, which means they had a level of t-TG antibodies higher than 100 U/ml. The mean t-TG level in the group of CD patients was 139 ± 162 U/ml. EMA was positive in 20 % of CD patients.

CD patients were divided into two groups based on t-TG levels with cut off value of 100 U/ml. Patients with low t-TG levels thus considered serologically negative had mean lumbar Z score of - 0.3 and mean left hip Z score of - 0.4 (n = 19) while serologically positive group had mean lumbar Z score of 0.0 and mean left hip Z score of - 0.3 (n = 15) (Figure 8). No statistically significant difference could be found in BMD between serologically positive and negative group with p values of 0.520 and 0.660 for lumbar spine Z scores and left hip Z scores, respectively. This was repeated after dividing the patients according to their EMA measurement. For EMA negative group mean lumbar Z score was - 0.1 and mean left hip Z score was - 0.4 (n = 26) while for EMA positive group mean lumbar spine Z score was - 0.4 and mean left hip Z score was - 0.3 (n = 7) (Figure 9). No significant difference was found in BMD between EMA positive and negative group with p = 0.391 for lumbar spine Z scores and p = 0.952 for left hip Z scores.

25

Figure 8: BMD in t-TG negative and positive CD patients.

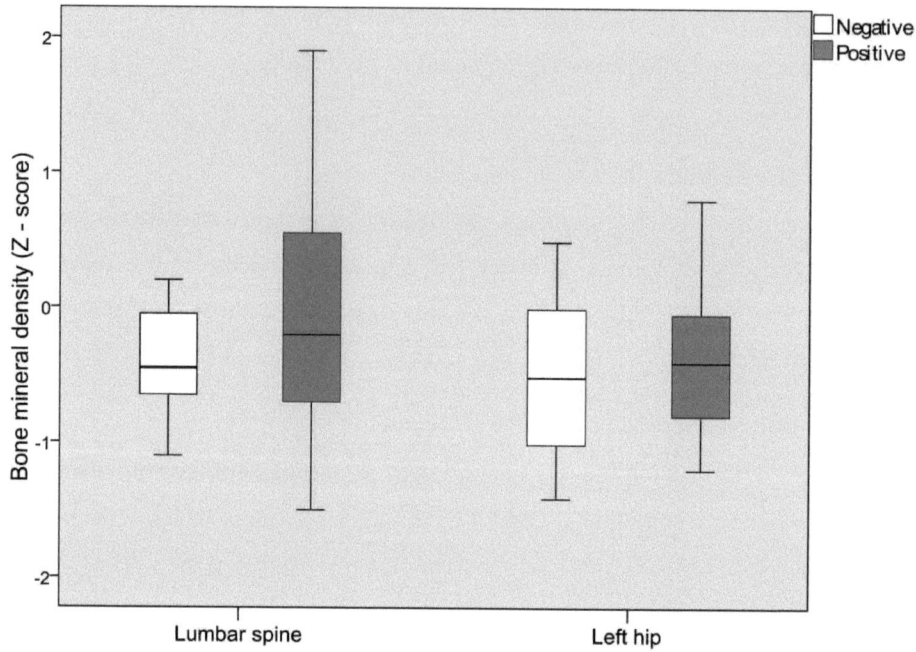

Figure 8 shows BMD measured at lumbar spine and left hip in serologically negative and positive CD patients, based on their t-TG. Serologically negative patients are shown in white bars, while serologically positive patients are shown in gray bars.

Figure 9: BMD in EMA negative and positive CD patients.

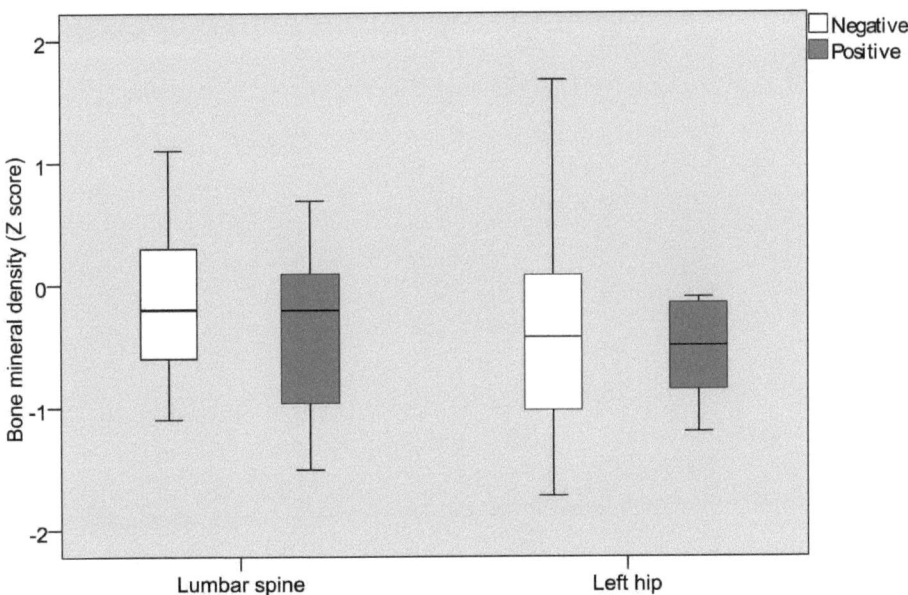

Figure 9 shows BMD measured at lumbar spine and left hip in serologically negative and positive CD patients, based on their EMA. Serologically negative patients are shown in white bars, while serologically positive patients are shown in gray bars.

Later, we focused on t-TG negative group of celiac disease patients (t-TG < 100 U/ml), who declared to comply with a strict GFD. Low levels of t-TG antibodies were considered to be a good indicator of diet compliance and therefore this group of patients had been actually serologically proven to be GFD compliant. Group of t-TG negative CD patients consisted of 22 patients (13 girls and 9 boys, with mean age 15 ± 2.6 years). Mean t-TG level of serologically negative group was 38 U/ml ± 27 U/ml. However, focused analysis revealed a marked negative correlation between BMD and serum t-TG levels where patients with lower t-TG levels achieved higher BMD scores than those closer to the upper limit of t-TG. Detailed analysis showed that the correlation between lumbar spine BMD and t-TG levels was statistically significant (R = - 0.5, p = 0.032) (Figure 10). Attempts were made to find a

27

correlation between left hip BMD, but the correlation did not reach statistical significance (p = 0.119) (Figure 11).

Figure 10: Lumbar spine BMD in serologically negative CD patients.

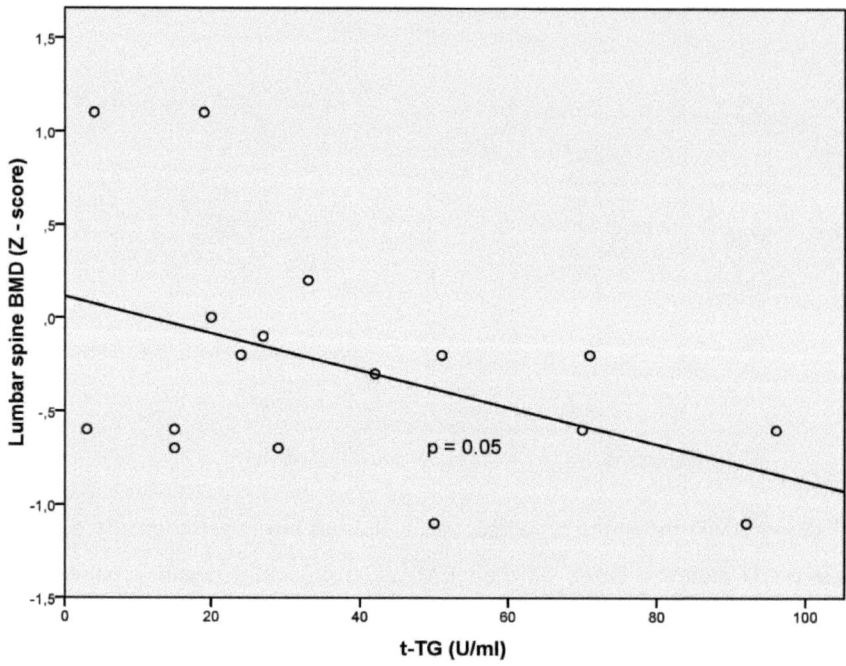

Figure represents correlation between BMD Z – scores measured at lumbar spine in serologically negative CD patients and t-TG values. The correlation is statistically significant.

Figure 11: Left hip BMD in serologically negative CD patients.

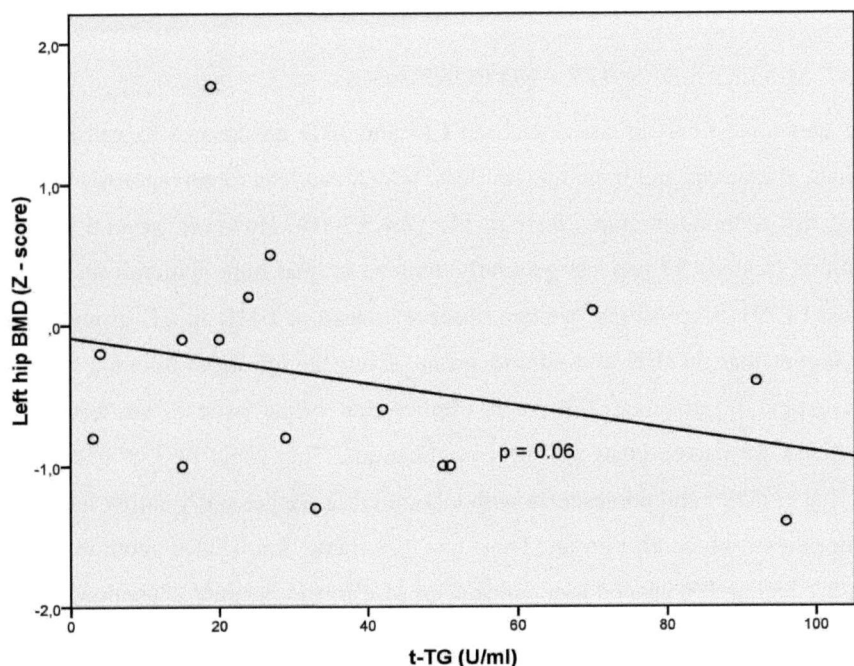

Figure represents correlation between BMD Z – scores measured at left hip in serologically negative CD patients and t-TG values. The correlation is not statistically significant.

5 DISCUSSION

5.1 BONE MINERAL DENSITY AND BONE AGE

Chronic gastrointestinal diseases, such as CD and IBD are known to cause bone metabolism alterations and bone mineral loss, which can lead to osteoporosis and an increased risk of bone fractures later in life (2,4,5,7-10). However, several studies reported that treated CD patients generally achieve normal bone mineralization and bone mass (4,79). Surprisingly, we can observe a trend of BMD in CD group being slightly higher than in IBD and control group. Even though the difference did not reach statistical significance, the result implies that celiac patients are not at an increased risk for osteoporosis and its complications. This could be explained with the fact that children and adolescents with CD on GFD are generally eating healthier than their peers from control group. They also have better knowledge about nutrition and healthy and well balanced diet, since a lot of effort is put into education of CD patients about their disease with a lot of emphasis on the importance of nutrition, physical activity and a healthy life style. However, Kautto et al. found that intake of nutrients in adolescents with CD was comparable with their healthy peers (80). Anyhow, these results are very promising. They show us that we are successful in preventing osteopenia, osteoporosis and decreasing the risk of bone fractures.

CD patients from our study were not given any vitamin or mineral supplements, so it seems that the strict GFD sufficed. However, bone health, including BMD in children with CD is usually impaired at the time of diagnosis, as described in many studies (3,4,5,74,79,81,82) but improves after the introduction of GFD, vitamin D and calcium supplementation (4,5,66,83-85). The study of Carvalho et al. found no difference in BMD in children with CD, but found lower BMD in adolescents with CD, compared to controls (86). However, in clinical practice the BMD and bone health are usually worse in children with CD than in their peers.

Low BMD is frequently detected in newly diagnosed children with IBD, particularly Crohn's disease (10). Mechanical properties of bone may worsen over time (84). In addition, height Z-scores may not improve with conventional IBD therapy (87) and muscle mass deficits may also persist, which can affect the accrual of bone mass, especially in patients with Crohn's disease (85,87). The risk of vertebral fractures may be increased, even without exposure to glucocorticoids (67). Our results also show that BMD Z scores in IBD patients in stable remission are comparable to those of the control. Our results suggest that we can be satisfied with the treatment of IBD patients, because normal BMD is usually more difficult to achieve in IBD patients than in CD patients (10,61). Results also support supplementation of IBD patients with vitamin D and calcium.

Our first hypothesis was therefore disproved: BMD in patients with CD and IBD was not significantly lower than BMD in healthy controls.

In addition, bone age was analyzed in all groups of children. Both groups of CD patients and control group had mean bone age slightly ahead of chronological age. This implies that both groups were appropriately developed according to the skeletal bone growth. While comparing both groups, no difference was found. This is consistent with previous results of BMD in different groups and confirms that their skeletal system is both chronologically well developed as well as sufficiently mineralized. While analyzing bone age, we found statistically significant correlation with lumbar spine BMD. Therefore, assesment of bone age in pediatric CD patients can be a fast and inexpensive tool for prediction of low BMD and thus related risks.

5.2 VITAMIN D

The results of our study show that serum vitamin D levels in children with CD or IBD were significantly lower than in the control group. This is in accordance with previous studies (5,62). In both CD and IBD patients the mean vitamin D levels were below reference values. This can be explained by malabsorption and gastrointestinal loss, which are the consequences of inflamed intestine, and possibly by a decreased sunlight exposure (62,75). Low dietary intake and poor compliance with vitamin D supplementation in IBD patients could also contribute to reduced vitamin D levels in the same group of patients.

When we compare the mean value of vitamin D in the control group to some other European countries, we observe lower concentrations of vitamin D (49.9 nmol/L vs. 57.1 nmol/L in other European countries) (88) which can be attributed to different diets (less foods rich in vitamin D, like oily fish), less exposure to sunlight or seasonal variations in vitamin D concentration.

The extent of vitamin D's role in bone mineralization in pediatric patients with chronic inflammatory gastrointestinal diseases has yet to be determined. A pediatric study of Sentongo et al. (89) reported no association between BMD and vitamin D status in children with Crohn's disease. It is not clear whether pre-existing vitamin D deficiency was the initiating event leading to disease severity, or vitamin D deficiency was the consequence of severe underlying illness (90).

It appears that the fall in vitamin D concentrations precedes lower BMD in our CD and IBD patients. Question remains, if and how long would it take for BMD to fall in these patients. Given that their vitamin D is lower than normal, vitamin D seems to have a minor effect on BMD in otherwise treated patients.

Previous studies reported the effect of vitamin D and calcium supplementation in BMD of children with specific chronic diseases. They reported increases in BMD of various skeletal sites with calcium and vitamin D supplementation, which was not observed without it (62). Adolescent with CD, who were treated from an early age

32

have BMD values similar to those of control (3). Moreover, an appropriate diet is very important in these patients, as naturally gluten-free products are often low in vitamin D, calcium, B vitamins, iron, zinc, magnesium, and fiber (89). Also, a study of dietary habits among children and adolescents in Slovenia revealed that dietary vitamin D intake was less than optimal and that calcium intake in boys was adequate, but bellow recommendations in girls (91). Therefore we advocate supplementation of pediatric patients with vitamin D and calcium, not only those with IBD, but also those with CD. Regular follow-ups are also important in ensuring patients follow their diet, prescribed medications and supplements.

Our second hypothesis was confirmed: values of vitamin D in patients with CD and IBD were significantly lower than vitamin D values in healthy controls.

Adolescents with IBD have unique issues such as poor medication compliance, growth failure, peer influence and risky behavior, which make managing teenage IBD patients more challenging (52). Similar challenges arise in children and adolescents with CD, especially if their symptoms are not prominent while not being on GFD. If they have no symptoms it is less likely that they will comply with strict GFD. Therefore it is critical to ensure and control appropriate treatment and diet compliance.

5.3 BODY COMPOSITION

At the measurements of body composition, girls had mean BF % values higher than boys, which is anthropometrically expected. We observed lower BF % in CD patients compared to IBD patients and controls which can be result of their disease and diet (92,93). BF % increases with implementation of GFD (93,94); however, the exact mechanism is not yet explained (95). Several other studies reported lower as well as higher values of BF % in children with IBD (76,96), which can also be seen in our results.

Girls had lower LBM which is expected due to their lower body weight and higher BF %. Girls with CD had lower LBM when compared to controls which is in concordance with previous study (93). Boys with CD had LBM values similar to boys with IBD and both were higher than boys in control group. Basically normal LBM values in boys with CD could again be explained with healthy diet and lifestyle.

Studies have shown positive correlation between body weight and BMD (97-99). It has been debated which of LBM or fat mass has more influence on bone stimulatory effect (100,101). Petit et al. suggest that bone strength is primarily determined by dynamic loads from muscle force and not static loads such as fat mass (102).

BIA is a lucrative method because of its ease of use, low costs and resources. The procedure takes only few minutes and it is non-invasive. Regarding its advantages, it would make sense to expand indications of BIA use. Some studies implicate, that body composition (and with this BF %) correlates with BMD (103).

Our results showed no statistically significant correlation between BF % and BMD or LBM and BMD in any of the groups, not even when subjects were divided in groups by sex. The use of BIA as additional diagnostic tool for determination of BMD was still described only in smaller number of studies. In those studies, one showed negative correlation between BF % and BMD in younger women, whereas other authors found positive correlation in pre- and postmenopausal women, and some found positive correlation in adult men and women (103-105). In one of more recent studies, positive correlation was found between BF % and BMD in prepubertal girls (97).

Our third hypothesis was disproved: BIA results did not correlate with BMD; therefore BIA is not a useful method in diagnosing lowered BMD.

BIA has potencial in clinical setting due to its practicality. However, the method will have to be studied more thoroughly. Body composition depends on many different factors and especially in pediatrics we have very heterogenous population, which differs by sex, age, height, weight, as well as level of development of various organ systems.

5.4 SEROLOGIC MARKERS

The only efficient treatment of CD thus far is a strict GFD. Therefore, a strict compliance to the diet is of great importance for the patients' wellbeing and should be evaluated by their physicians regularly (2,5,7). Serological markers (both t-TG and EMA) were found to be good markers for the objective determination of the patients` compliance with GFD (12,35). Studies outline both t-TG and EMA to be useful tool for both diagnosis of CD and follow-up (12,35,106,107). Percentage of serologically positive CD patients was 44 % and 20 % for t-TG and EMA, respectively. The percentage of serologically positive CD patients seems high, given the fact that they were all self-declared to be fully aware and adherent to the GFD.

Furthermore, we investigated the effect of elevated t-TG levels on BMD in children and adolescents with CD. However, no statistically significant difference was found when comparing BMD between the groups with t-TG positive and t-TG negative levels, which could be a result of relatively small sample of patients. The same analysis was repeated after separating CD patients in groups of EMA positive and EMA negative patients. However, no significant difference was found. Further studies are needed with larger groups of patients.

We hypothesized there should be a correlation between t-TG and BMD since serological markers are well accepted tool for monitoring the disease and there are plenty of evidence regarding the effect of CD on BMD (1,2,5,12,106,108). Since there is evidence that decreased concentrations of t-TG antibodies are significantly associated with the degree of compliance with the GFD, correlation between t-TG and BMD is also expected (37,38). To our best knowledge, not many studies had focused directly on that particular relation, yet Kocsis et al. had mentioned a correlation between those two in his observation of a single celiac centre (109).

It is reasonable to expect the difference in BMD between the groups of patients on a strict GFD and those who are not on GFD. Patients who were complying with the strict GFD and were checked regularly by their pediatrician (with both clinical examination and laboratory studies), were therefore considered as being appropriately treated and expected to be at equally low risk for reduced BMD. However, when analyzing the results we found a difference in BMD within the group of children that were considered to be on a strict GFD by self-reported dietary history, and who also had levels of t-TG within the normal range. We discovered that there was a significant difference among the patients who were considered as being well treated and appropriately complying with GFD. Statistically significant correlation was found between BMD and the levels of t-TG. Those with low t-TG levels had significantly better BMD than those with higher t-TG levels while still being low enough to be considered serologically negative (p = 0.032). Our results are in agreement with Kocsis' study, in which a correlation has been established between BMD and t-TG (109). Agardh's study showed similar results yet with different antibodies, while Margoni's study stated that no biochemical marker is capable of predicting an abnormal BMD (84,110). No other study that we know of focused on a group of t-TG negative patients and presented t-TG as a tool for detecting a decreased BMD in CD patients who were considered well treated.

This raises several questions regarding the appropriate definition of reference values, as well as the use of serological markers as an objective tool for evaluating treatment success. It shows that not merely the diet itself, but also the strictness of the diet is important and the consequences can be reflected on the bone mineral density. The risk of all future complications of CD, not merely risk of bone fractures, may very likely be related to the strictness of the diet in a much greater way than it was previously suspected. The results of our study should encourage all physicians dealing with celiac disease to advise their patients to follow a strict gluten-free diet as much as possible. Physicians should not have the reference values of serological markers as the goal of the treatment but rather tend to achieve the diet as strict as possible and have the serological markers the lowest possible. Only in that way can we be certain that patients are getting the best possible treatment.

6 CONCLUSION

Early diagnosis and effective treatment are of utmost importance in preventing pediatric patient's suboptimal peak bone mass, osteoporosis and increased risk of fracture in the future. Satisfactory BMD in our CD and IBD patients warrant strict compliance with GFD in CD and necessity of good disease control in IBD patients. Even within the group of patients with CD, who declared to be on a strict GFD, we found a spectrum of strictness of the diet which influenced their BMD accordingly. This finding raises the importance of a strict gluten free diet. We also found low levels of vitamin D in CD and IBD patients and this supports our supplementation of our patients with vitamin D and calcium. Even though we did not confirm applicability of BIA in determining changes in BMD, due to its practicalities, further studies are needed to determine its indications and position in the diagnostics of lowered BMD.

7 REFERENCES

1. Larussa T, Suraci E, Nazionale I, Abenavoli L, Imeneo M, Luzza F. Bone mineralization in celiac disease. Gastroenterol Res Pract. 2012;2012:198025.

2. Kalayci AG, Kansu A, Girgin N, Kucuk O, Aras G. Bone mineral density and importance of a gluten-free diet in patients with celiac disease in childhood. Pediatrics. 2001;108(5):E89.

3. Kavak US, Yüce A, Koçak N, Demir H, Saltik IN, Gürakan F, et al. Bone mineral density in children with untreated and treated celiac disease. J Pediatr Gastroenterol Nutr. 2003;37(4):434-6.

4. Heyman R, Guggenbuhl P, Corbel A, Bridoux-Henno L, Tourtelier Y, Balençon-Morival M, et al. Effect of a gluten-free diet on bone mineral density in children with celiac disease. Gastroenterol Clin Biol. 2009;33(2):109-14.

5. Blazina S, Bratanic N, Campa AS, Blagus R, Orel R. Bone mineral density and importance of strict gluten-free diet in children and adolescents with celiac disease. Bone. 2010;47(3):598-603.

6. Tau C, Mautalen C, De Rosa S, Roca A, Valenzuela X. Bone mineral density in children with celiac disease. Effect of a Gluten-free diet. Eur J Clin Nutr. 2006;60(3):358-63.

7. Boot AM, Bouquet J, Krenning EP, de Muinck Keizer-Schrama SM. Bone mineral density and nutritional status in children with chronic inflammatory bowel disease. Gut 1998;42(2):188-194.

8. Paganelli M, Albanese C, Borrelli O, Civitelli F, Canitano N, Viola F et al. Inflammation is the main determinant of low bone mineral density in pediatric inflammatory bowel disease. Inflamm Bowel Dis 2007;13(4):416-423.

9. Ali T, Lam D, Bronze MS, Humphrey MB. Osteoporosis in inflammatory bowel disease. Am J Med 2009;122(7):599-604.

10. Sylvester FA, Wyzga N, Hyams JS, Davis PM, Lerer T, Vance K et al. Natural history of bone metabolism and bone mineral density in children with inflammatory bowel disease. Inflamm Bowel Dis 2007;13(1):42-50.

11. Sentongo TA, Semeao EJ, Piccoli DA, Stallings VA, Zemel BS. Growth, body composition, and nutritional status in children and adolescents with Crohn's disease. J Pediatr Gastroenterol Nutr. 2000 Jul;31(1):33-40

12. Husby S, Koletzko S, Korponay-Szabó IR, Mearin ML, Phillips A, Shamir R, et al.; ESPGHAN Working Group on Coeliac Disease Diagnosis; ESPGHAN Gastroenterology Committee; European Society for Pediatric Gastroenterology, Hepatology, and Nutrition. European Society for Pediatric Gastroenterology, Hepatology, and Nutrition guidelines for the diagnosis of coeliac disease. J Pediatr Gastroenterol Nutr. 2012;54(1):136-60.

13. Malamut G, Cellier C. Celiac disease. Rev Med Interne. 2010;31(6):428-33.

14. Greco L, Timpone L, Abkari A, Abu-Zekry M, Attard T, Bouguerrà F, et al. Burden of celiac disease in the Mediterranean area. World J Gastroenterol. 2011;17(45):4971-8.

15. Lohi S, Mustalahti K, Kaukinen K, Laurila K, Collin P, Rissanen H, et al. Increasing prevalence of coeliac disease over time. Aliment Pharmacol Ther. 2007;26(9):1217-25.

16: Tucci F, Astarita L, Abkari A, Abu-Zekry M, Attard T, Ben Hariz M, Bilbao JR, Boudraa G, Boukthir S, Costa S, Djurisic V, Hugot JP, Irastorza I, Kansu A, Kolaček S, Magazzù G, Mičetić-Turk D, Misak Z, Roma E, Rossi P, Terzic S, Velmishi V, Arcidiaco C, Auricchio R, Greco L. Celiac disease in the Mediterranean area. BMC Gastroenterol. 2014 Feb 11;14:24

17. Catassi C, Cobellis G. Coeliac disease epidemiology is alive and kicking, especially in the developing world. Dig Liver Dis. 2007;39(10):908-10.

18. Schuppan D, Hahn EG. Gluten and the gut – lessons for immune regulation. Science 2002;297:2218–20.

19. Holtmeier W, Caspary WF. Celiac disease. Orphanet J Rare Dis. 2006;1:3.

20. Sapone A, Bai JC, Ciacci C, Dolinsek J, Green PH, Hadjivassiliou M, et al. Spectrum of gluten-related disorders: consensus on new nomenclature and classification. BMC Med. 2012;10:13.

21. Ferretti G, Bacchetti T, Masciangelo S, Saturni L. Celiac disease, inflammation and oxidative damage: a nutrigenetic approach. Nutrients. 2012;4(4):243-57.

22. Ravikumara M, Tuthill DP, Jenkins HR. The changing clinical presentation of coeliac disease. Arch Dis Child. 2006;91(12):969-71.

23. Wahab PJ, Meijer JW, Dumitra D, Goerres MS, Mulder CJ. Coeliac disease: more than villous atrophy. Rom J Gastroenterol. 2002;11(2):121-7.

24. Turner J, Pellerin G, Mager D. Prevalence of metabolic bone disease in children with celiac disease is independent of symptoms at diagnosis. J Pediatr Gastroenterol Nutr. 2009;49(5):589-93.

25. Capriles VD, Martini LA, Arêas JA. Metabolic osteopathy in celiac disease: importance of a gluten-free diet. Nutr Rev. 2009;67(10):599-606.

26. Dolinsek J, Urlep D, Karell K, Partanen J, Micetić-Turk D. The prevalence of celiac disease among family members of celiac disease patients. Wien Klin Wochenschr. 2004;116 Suppl 2:8-12.

27. Tjon JM, van Bergen J, Koning F. Celiac disease: how complicated can it get? Immunogenetics. 2010;62(10):641-51.

28: Szałowska-Woźniak DA, Bąk-Romaniszyn L, Cywińska-Bernas A, Zeman K. Evaluation of HLA-DQ2/DQ8 genotype in patients with celiac disease hospitalised in 2012 at the Department of Paediatrics. Prz Gastroenterol. 2014;9(1):32-7.

29. Micetić-Turk D, Umek-Bradac S, Dolinsek J, Gorenjak M, Turk Z, Skalicky M. Ultrasonographic assessment of celiac disease in children: comparison with antiendomysium antibodies and histology. Wien Klin Wochenschr. 2001;113(3):2-31.

30: Bhattacharya M, Lomash A, Sakhuja P, Dubey AP, Kapoor S. Clinical and histopathological correlation of duodenal biopsy with IgA anti-tissue transglutaminase titers in children with celiac disease. Indian J Gastroenterol. 2014 May 24.

31. Kav T, Sivri B. Is enteroscopy necessary for diagnosis of celiac disease? World J Gastroenterol. 2012;18(31):4095-101.

32. Esposito C, Caputo I, Troncone R. New therapeutic strategies for coeliac disease: tissue transglutaminase as a target. Curr Med Chem. 2007;14(24):2572-80.

33. Kurppa K, Räsänen T, Collin P, Iltanen S, Huhtala H, et al. Endomysial antibodies predict celiac disease irrespective of the titers or clinical presentation. World J Gastroenterol. 2012;18(20):2511-6.

34: Pelkowski TD, Viera AJ. Celiac disease: diagnosis and management. Am Fam Physician. 2014 Jan 15;89(2):99-105.

35. Setty M, Hormaza L, Guandalini S. Celiac disease: risk assessment, diagnosis, and monitoring. Mol Diagn Ther. 2008;12(5):289-98.

36. Di Sabatino A, Vanoli A, Giuffrida P, Luinetti O, Solcia E, Corazza GR. The function of tissue transglutaminase in celiac disease. Autoimmun Rev. 2012 Aug;11(10):746-53.

37. Nachman F, Sugai E, Vázquez H, González A, Andrenacci P, et al. Serological tests for celiac disease as indicators of long-term compliance with the gluten-free diet. Eur J Gastroenterol Hepatol. 2011 Jun;23(6):473-80.

38. Sugai E, Nachman F, Váquez H, González A, Andrenacci P, et al. Dynamics of celiac disease-specific serology after initiation of a gluten-free diet and use in the assessment of compliance with treatment. Dig Liver Dis. 2010 May;42(5):352-8.

39. Zanini B, Lanzarotto F, Mora A, Bertolazzi S, Turini D, et al. Five year time course of celiac disease serology during gluten free diet: results of a community based "CD-Watch" program. Dig Liver Dis. 2010 Dec;42(12):865-70.

40. Dipper CR, Maitra S, Thomas R, Lamb CA, McLean-Tooke AP, et al. Anti-tissue transglutaminase antibodies in the follow-up of adult coeliac disease. Aliment Pharmacol Ther. 2009 Aug;30(3):236-44.

41. Hill ID, Dirks MH, Liptak GS, Colletti RB, Fasano A, Guandalini S, et al. North American Society for Pediatric Gastroenterology, Hepatology and Nutrition. Guideline for the diagnosis and treatment of celiac disease in children: recommendations of the North American Society for Pediatric Gastroenterology, Hepatology and Nutrition. J Pediatr Gastroenterol Nutr. 2005;40(1):1-19.

42: Caruso R, Pallone F, Stasi E, Romeo S, Monteleone G. Appropriate nutrient supplementation in celiac disease. Ann Med. 2013 Dec;45(8):522-31.

43: Kurppa K, Paavola A, Collin P, Sievänen H, Laurila K, Huhtala H, Päivi Saavalainen, Mäki M, Kaukinen K. Benefits of a Gluten-free diet for Asymptomatic Patients with Serologic Markers of Celiac Disease. Gastroenterology. 2014 May 13.pii: S0016-5085(14)00609-X.

44. Catassi C, Fabiani E, Iacono G, D'Agate C, Francavilla R, Biagi F, et al. A prospective, double-blind, placebo-controlled trial to establish a safe gluten threshold for patients with celiac disease. Am J Clin Nutr. 2007;85(1):160-6.

45. Codex alimentarius (2008) Codex standard for foods for special dietary use for persons intolerant to gluten—Codex Stan 118-1979.

46. Prevention and management of osteoporosis: Report of a WHO Scientific Group. WHO Scientific Group on the Prevention and Management of Osteoporosis 2000: Geneva, Switzerland; 2003.

47. Košnik M, Mrevlje F, Štajer D, editors. Interna medicina. Ljubljana: Littera Picta; 2011.

48. Kliegman RM, Behrman RE, Jenson HB, Stanton B. Nelson Textbook of Pediatrics. 19th ed. Philadelphia: Elsevier/Saunders; 2011.

49. Matricon J, Barnich N, Ardid D. Immunopathogenesis of inflammatory bowel disease. Self Nonself. 2010 Oct;1(4):299-309.

50) Gokhaler R. Crohn's disease and indeterminate colitis. Chapter 21 in Essential pediatric gastroenterology, hepatohology, and nutrition. 2005: 251-60.

51. Sciaudone G, Di Stazio C, Limongelli P, Guadagni I, Pellino G, Riegler G, et al. Treatment of complex perianal fistulas in Crohn disease: infliximab, surgery or combined approach. Can J Surg. 2010;53(5):299-304.

52. Lu Y, Markowitz J. Inflammatory bowel disease in adolescents: what problems does it pose? World J Gastroenterol. 2011;17(22):2691-5.

53. Zanchi C, Di Leo G, Ronfani L, Martelossi S, Not T, Ventura A. Bone metabolism in celiac disease. J Pediatr. 2008;153(2):262-5.

54. Molteni N, Bardella MT, Vezzoli G, Pozzoli E, Bianchi P. Intestinal calcium absorption as shown by stable strontium test in celiac disease before and after gluten-free diet. Am J Gastroenterol. 1995;90(11):2025-8.

55. Szathmári M, Tulassay T, Arató A, Bodánszky H, Szabó A, Tulassay Z. Bone mineral content and density in asymptomatic children with coeliac disease on a gluten-free diet. Eur J Gastroenterol Hepatol 2001;13(4):419-424.

56. Viswanathan A, Sylvester FA. Chronic pediatric inflammatory diseases: effects on bone. Rev Endocr Metab Disord 2008;9(2):107-122.

57. Sánchez MI, Mohaidle A, Baistrocchi A, Matoso D, Vázquez H, González A, et al. Risk of fracture in celiac disease: gender, dietary compliance, or both? World J Gastroenterol. 2011;17(25):3035-42.

58. Katz S, Weinerman S. Osteoporosis and gastrointestinal disease. Gastroenterol Hepatol. 2010;6(8):506-17.

59. Mulder CJ, Cardile AP, Dickert J. Celiac disease presenting as severe osteopenia. Hawaii Med J. 2011;70(11):242-4.

60. Mora S, Weber G, Barera G, Bellini A, Pasolini D, Prinster C et al. Effect of gluten-free diet on bone mineral content in growing patients with celiac disease. Am J Clin Nutr 1993;57(2):224-228.

61. Lacativa PG, Farias ML. Osteoporosis and inflammation. Arq Bras Endocrinol Metabol 2010;54(2):123-32.

62. Pappa HM, Grand RJ, Gordon CM. Report on the vitamin D status of adult and pediatric patients with inflammatory bowel disease and its significance for bone health and disease. Inflamm Bowel Dis 2006;12(12):1162-1174.

63. Miheller P, Lorinczy K, Lakatos PL. Clinical relevance of changes in bone metabolism in inflammatory bowel disease. World J Gastroenterol 2010;16(44):5536-5542.

64. Laakso S, Valta H, Verkasalo M, Toiviainen-Salo S, Mäkitie O. Compromised Peak Bone Mass in Patients with Inflammatory Bowel Disease-A Prospective Study. J Pediatr. 2014 Mar 17.

65. Legido J, Gisbert JP, Pajares JM, Maté J. Bone metabolism changes in patients with inflammatory bowel disease. Rev Esp Enferm Dig 2005;97(11):815-829.

66. Bernstein CN, Leslie WD. The pathophysiology of bone disease in gastrointestinal disease. Eur J Gastroenterol Hepatol 2003;15(8):857-564.

67. Wong SC, Catto-Smith AG, Zacharin M. Pathological fractures in paediatric patients with inflammatory bowel disease. Eur J Pediatr. 2014 Feb;173(2):141-51.

68. Boyce BF, Xing L. The RANKL/RANK/OPG pathway. Curr Osteoporos Rep 2007;5(3):98-104.

69. Przemioslo RT, Kontakou M, Nobili V, Ciclitira PJ. Raised pro-inflammatory cytokines interleukin 6 and tumour necrosis factor alpha in coeliac disease mucosa detected by immunohistochemistry. Gut 1994;35(10):1398-1403.

70. Westerholm-Ormio M, Garioch J, Ketola I, Savilahti E. Inflammatory cytokines in small intestinal mucosa of patients with potential coeliac disease. Clin Exp Immunol 2002;128(1):94-101.

71. Bernstein CN. Inflammatory bowel diseases as secondary causes of osteoporosis. Curr Osteoporos Rep 2006;4(3):116-123.

72. El-Matary W, Sikora S, Spady D. Bone mineral density, vitamin D, and disease activity in children newly diagnosed with inflammatory bowel disease. Dig Dis Sci 2011;56(3):825-829.

73. Mager DR, Qiao J, Turner J. Vitamin D and K status influences bone mineral density and bone accrual in children and adolescents with celiac disease. Eur J Clin Nutr 2012;66(4):488-495.

74. Lerner A, Shapira Y, Agmon-Levin N, Pacht A, Ben-Ami Shor D, López HM, et al. The clinical significance of 25OH-Vitamin D status in celiac disease. Clin Rev Allergy Immunol 2012;42(3):322-330.

46

75. Pappa HM, Gordon CM, Saslowsky TM, Zholudev A, Horr B, Shih MC, et al. Vitamin D status in children and young adults with inflammatory bowel disease. Pediatrics 2006;118(5):1950-1961.

76. Wiskin AE, Wootton SA, Hunt TM, Cornelius VR, Afzal NA, Jackson AA et al. Body composition in childhood inflammatory bowel disease. Clin Nutr 2011;30(1):112-115.

77. Samasca G, Iancu M, Farcau D, Butnariu A, Pop T, et al. IgA anti-tissue transglutaminase antibodies, first line in the diagnosis of celiac disease. Clin Lab. 2011;57(9-10):695-701.

78. Carroccio A, Iacono G, Di Prima L, Pirrone G, Cavataio F, et al. Antiendomysium antibodies assay in the culture medium of intestinal mucosa: an accurate method for celiac disease diagnosis. Eur J Gastroenterol Hepatol. 2011;23(11):1018-23.

79. Mora S, Barera G, Ricotti A, Weber G, Bianchi C, Chiumello G. Reversal of low bone density with a gluten-free diet in children and adolescents with celiac disease. Am J Clin Nutr 1998;67(3):477-481.

80. Kautto E, Ivarsson A, Norström F, Högberg L, Carlsson A, Hörnell A. Nutrient intake in adolescent girls and boys diagnosed with coeliac disease at an early age is mostly comparable to their non-coeliac contemporaries. J Hum Nutr Diet. 2014 Feb;27(1):41-53.

81. Mora S, Barera G, Beccio S, Menni L, Proverbio MC, Bianchi C et al. A prospective, longitudinal study of the long-term effect of treatment on bone density in children with celiac disease. J Pediatr 2001;139(4):516-521.

82. Barera G, Beccio S, Proverbio MC, Mora S. Longitudinal changes in bone metabolism and bone mineral content in children with celiac disease during consumption of a gluten-free diet. Am J Clin Nutr 2004;79(1):148-154.

83. Jatla M, Zemel BS, Bierly P, Verma R. Bone mineral content deficits of the spine and whole body in children at time of diagnosis with celiac disease. J Pediatr Gastroenterol Nutr 2009;48(2):175-180.

84. Margoni D, Chouliaras G, Duscas G, Voskaki I, Voutsas N, Papadopoulou A et al. Bone health in children with celiac disease assessed by dual x-ray absorptiometry: effect of gluten-free diet and predictive value of serum biochemical indices. J Pediatr Gastroenterol Nutr 2012;54(5):680-684.

85. Dubner SE, Shults J, Baldassano RN, Zemel BS, Thayu M, Burnham JM et al. Longitudinal assessment of bone density and structure in an incident cohort of children with Crohn's disease. Gastroenterology 2009;136(1):123-130.

86. Carvalho CN, Sdepanian VL, de Morais MB, Fagundes Neto U. (Celiac disease under treatment: evaluation of bone mineral density). J Pediatr (Rio J) 2003;79(4):303-308.

87. Pfefferkorn M, Burke G, Griffiths A, Markowitz J, Rosh J, Mack D et al. Growth abnormalities persist in newly diagnosed children with crohn disease despite current treatment paradigms. J Pediatr Gastroenterol Nutr 2009;48(2):168-174.

88. González-Gross M, Valtueña J, Breidenassel C, Moreno LA, Ferrari M, Kersting M et al. Vitamin D status among adolescents in Europe: the Healthy Lifestyle in Europe by Nutrition in Adolescence study. Br J Nutr 2012;107(5):755-764.

89. Sentongo TA, Semaeo EJ, Stettler N, Piccoli DA, Stallings VA, Zemel BS. Vitamin D status in children, adolescents, and young adults with Crohn disease. Am J Clin Nutr 2002;76(5):1077-1081.

90. Raman M, Milestone AN, Walters JR, Hart AL, Ghosh S. Vitamin D and gastrointestinal diseases: inflammatory bowel disease and colorectal cancer. Therap Adv Gastroenterol 2011;4(1):49-62.

91. Fidler Mis N, Kobe H, Stimec M. Dietary intake of macro- and micronutrients in slovenian adolescents: comparison with reference values. Ann Nutr Metab 2012;61(4):305-313.

92. Duerksen DR, Leslie WD. Longitudinal evaluation of bone mineral density and body composition in patients with positive celiac serology. J Clin Densitom 2011;14(4):478-483.

93. Barera G, Mora S, Brambilla P, Ricotti A, Menni L, Beccio S, et al. Body composition in children with celiac disease and the effects of a gluten-free diet: a prospective case-control study. Am J Clin Nutr 2000;72(1):71-75.

94. Carbone MC, Pitzalis G, Ferri M, Nenna R, Thanasi E, Andreoli A, De Lorenzo A, Bonamico M. Body composition in coeliac disease adolescents on a gluten-free diet: a longitudinal study. Acta Diabetol. 2003 Oct;40 Suppl 1:S171-3.

95. Rea F, Polito C, Marotta A, Di Toro A, Iovene A, Collini R, Rea L, Sessa G. Restoration of body composition in celiac children after one year of gluten-free diet. J Pediatr Gastroenterol Nutr. 1996 Nov;23(4):408-12.

96. Sylvester FA, Leopold S, Lincoln M, Hyams JS, Griffiths AM, Lerer T. A two-year longitudinal study of persistent lean tissue deficits in children with Crohn's disease. Clin Gastroenterol Hepatol. 2009;7(4):452-5.

97. Rhie YJ, Lee KH, Chung SC, Kim HS, Kim DH. Effects of body composition, leptin, and adiponectin on bone mineral density in prepubertal girls. J Korean Med Sci. 2010;25(8):1187-90.

98. Reid IR. Relationships among body mass, its components, and bone. Bone 2002;31:547-55.

99. Zemel B. Bone mineral accretion and its relationship to growth, sexual maturation and body composition during childhood and adolescence. World Rev Nutr Diet. 2013;106:39-45.

100. Van Langendonck L, Claessens AL, Lefevre J, Thomis M, Philippaerts R, Delvaux K, Lysens R, Vanden Eynde B, Beunen G. Association between bone mineral density (DXA), body structure, and body composition in middle-aged men. Am J Hum Biol 2002;14:735-42.

101. Glauber HS, Vollmer WM, Nevitt MC, Ensrud KE, Orwoll ES. Body weight versus body fat distribution, adiposity, and frame size as predictors of bone density. J Clin Endocrinol Metab 1995;80:1118-23.

102. Petit MA, Beck TJ, Shults J, Zemel BS, Foster BJ, Leonard MB. Proximal femur bone geometry is appropriately adapted to lean mass in overweight children and adolescents. Bone 2005;36:568-576.

103. Ngai HH, Cheung CL, Yao TJ, Kung AW. Bioimpedance: can its addition to simple clinical criteria enhance the diagnosis of osteoporosis? J Bone Miner Metab 2009;27(3):372-378.

104. Arimatsu M, Kitano T, Kitano N, Inomoto T, Shono M, Futatsuka M. Correlation between forearm bone mineral density and body composition in Japanese females aged 18-40 years. Environ Health Prev Med. 2005;10(3):144-9.

105. Zhao HY, Liu JM, Ning G, Zhang LZ, Xu MY, Chen JL. The relationship between body composition measured with bioelectric impedance analysis and bone mass in female. Zhonghua Nei Ke Za Zhi. 2004;43(7):506-9.

106. Mohaidle A, Mella JM, Pereyra L, Luna P, Fischer C, et al. Role of antibodies in celiac disease after one year of treatment to predict the adherence to gluten-free diet. Acta Gastroenterol Latinoam. 2011 Mar;41(1):23-8.

107: Lakos G, Norman GL, Mahler M, Martis P, Bentow C, Santora D, Fasano A. Analytical and clinical comparison of two fully automated immunoassay systems for the diagnosis of celiac disease. J Immunol Res. 2014;2014:371263.

108. Hogen Esch CE, Wolters VM, Gerritsen SA, Putter H, von Blomberg BM, et al. Specific celiac disease antibodies in children on a gluten-free diet. Pediatrics. 2011;128(3):547-52.

109. Kocsis D, Miheller P, Lőrinczy K, Herszényi L, Tulassay Z, et al. Coeliac disease in a 15-year period of observation (1997 and 2011) in a Hungarian referral centre. Eur J Intern Med. 2013;24(5):461-7.

110. Agardh D, Björck S, Agardh CD, Lidfeldt J. Coeliac disease-specific tissue transglutaminase autoantibodies are associated with osteoporosis and related fractures in middle-aged women. Scand J Gastroenterol. 2009;44(5):571-8.

8 ACKNOWLEDGEMENTS

The authors thank the children and adolescents who participated and their parents for their consent.

The authors are indebted to dr. Jernej Dolinšek and Maja Šikić Pogačar for their help during the study and for revision of manuscript.

We would like to thank the staff of Pediatric Clinic of University Medical Centre Maribor as well as the staff of Endocrinology and Diabetics Department, the staff of Department of Laboratory Diagnostics and the staff of Department of Radiology at University Medical Centre Maribor for all the help in this research.

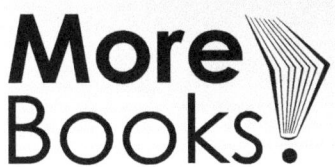
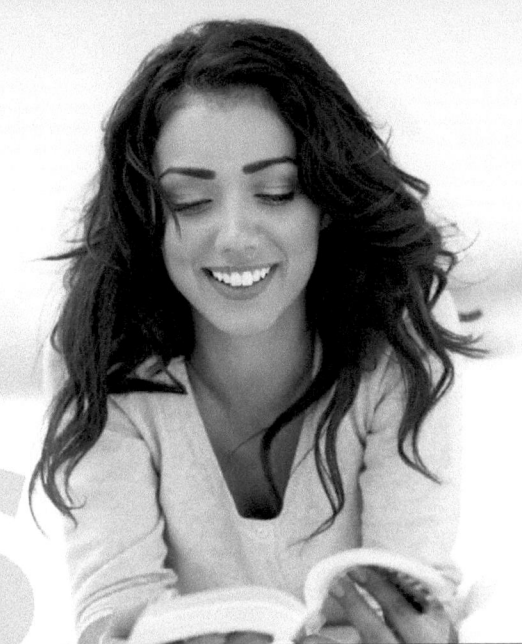
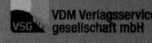

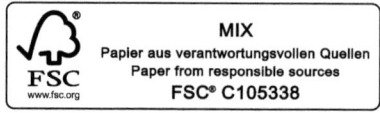
Printed by Books on Demand GmbH, Norderstedt / Germany